Train Your Taste

To

Trim Your Waist

By

Drew Canole

Free Reader Bonus

Only Available To You

As A Thank You For Reading

"Train Your Taste To Trim Your Waist."

Visit

http://trainyourtaste.com/reader-bonus

See Drew Canole's #1 Best Seller on Amazon:

"Juicing Recipes For Vitality And Health"

https://www.amazon.com/dp/B007DDQYCU

Forward By A Transformation Client Of Drew Canole

Have you ever picked up a book that you were excited to read and half way through you just stopped because the author droned on about pointless material until you lost interest and set it aside?

That will not happen here. This is a **refreshingly short book**, which is more like a "call to action." You are about to get Drew Canole's proven protocol for training your taste buds to enjoy healthy food.

This will cause you to eat the way you should be eating. It will clear the path for fat-loss and physical transformation, which has been blocked by your little taste buds. And you'll learn that they aren't necessarily your "buds" at all.

I know this because I hired the author of this book, Drew Canole, to be my personal transformation coach. Investing enough money to take a luxurious week-long trip to Maui makes you sit up and pay attention to what you're being told, at least it did for me.

I hired him to get me eating right, exercising and staying motivated to achieve my goals. This is Drew's gift. He believes in you, even when you don't believe in yourself and he does more than motivate you to succeed, he inspires you to transform your life.

I saw the successful transformations that others achieved with his programs and I wanted the same thing. I was far from obese, but I was tired, flabby, injury-prone and was getting sick more than I thought normal.

Drew Canole's program was the catalyst to me finally achieving six pack abs after thirty-seven years of trying. That may sound superficial, but it was one thing that motivated me every day and depressed me that no matter how hard I tried on my own, I couldn't make them materialize.

Working out never gave me the results I wanted. Long hours of cardio and weights were cancelled out by my sweet tooth and love of chips, salsa and sandwiches. "Abs are made in the kitchen" was the mantra Drew made me repeat until I was blue in the face. But it didn't matter because every time I tried to cook healthy or order the healthy option at the restaurant, that devil on my shoulder (or rather the devils on my tongue) would convince me to splurge.

I would tell myself: "life is too short not to enjoy the food you're eating." Drew said he agreed, and that the key was to learn how to enjoy the foods that will burn the belly fat off of me without ever feeling like I'm sacrificing flavor.

"You snack on lifeless, processed crap" he told me, "while I snack on sunshine. The food I eat is food I love and it nourishes my body, my soul and my mind. In fact, I crave the food you avoid. And I can teach you to do the same thing. That is…if you want it bad enough."

Drew followed through on his promise and to this day I not only feel better, have more energy and like what I see in the mirror, but I crave broccoli! Lean meats and fresh veggies are more satisfying than any of the sugary, fat-loaded food of which I used to be addicted.

Drew trained my taste, which helped to trim my waist, and he did it in less than a month. The information in this book is pulled directly from the comprehensive transformation and training protocol he put me through, the one I invested thousands of dollars to receive.

This plan will only work however, if you read it. This is the reason it's not a fluff-filled book with several hundred pages of theories, stories and anecdotes. Most people (myself included) have multiple half-finished books lying around that we purchased with good intentions but failed to get to the end. That should not be a problem with this book

Just like any diet or exercise plan, the best one for you is the one you actually DO. This is no different.

-Brad Costanzo, personal transformation client of Drew Canole

Table of Contents

Chapter 1: Why does everything that's bad for me taste so good?"
....1

Chapter 2: Abs Are Made In The Kitchen...................................9

Chapter 3: Why You Probably Aren't Eating
Right . . . Right Now 13

Chapter 4: Your Taste Buds Are Traitors! 21

Chapter 5: How Susan Trained Her Taste Buds........................25

Chapter 6: Old Dogs Mastering New Tricks 27

Chapter 7: How To Train Your Taste To Trim Your Waist 31

Chapter 8: Day 22 63

Chapter 9: Let's Recap The Protocol......................................81

Chapter 10: (((The Ripple Effect)))......................................83

RESOURCES...89

Chapter 1:

"Why does everything that's bad for me taste so good?"

Have you ever asked yourself the question above? Almost every one of us has. But consider the following.

What If healthy-food tasted delicious and fried foods made us cringe?

What if fresh steamed veggies made our mouths water?

What if a glass of freshly squeezed vegetable-juice tasted much better than a Coke or Pepsi?

And what if children actually begged for broccoli instead of cookies? (Ok, maybe *this* one is wishful thinking).

If these "what if's" were a reality for you, if you really did gravitate toward the healthiest option naturally, how difficult would it then be to lose that extra fat around your midsection?

How much easier would it be to watch weight melt off of you and finally achieve the body of your dreams, or the body of your youth, for that matter?

What if you loved the food that loves you back? What if you craved the food that makes your body run like the finely tuned machine it really is? You would never be on a "diet" and you would never be stressed out about avoiding the food you loved.

It may sound like wishful thinking, only true in fantasies. But it can be real for you.

I'm going to give you a step-by-step method to lose inches around your waist, drop fat from your body, and heal yourself from the inside out.

You will find yourself actually craving the most nourishing foods that you know you should eat—the kind of food that gives you energy and removes unwanted weight. The junky, processed foods that have a death grip on your taste buds will soon be just an occasional treat you give yourself instead of a warden keeping your weight loss plans locked up.

You are going to discover how your traitorous and unruly taste buds are literally ruining your dreams of a flat belly, six-pack abs, or just a trim, firm waistline. Like an unruly child throwing temper tantrums or an untrained dog who refuses to obey, as much as you love them they can make your life miserable until you get them under control.

Training your taste buds is the key to transforming a laborious and miserable "diet" into an effortlessly healthy and rewarding lifestyle that you enjoy.

These are the results you'll see:

Once your taste is trained, choosing the healthy option on the menu will become second nature, cooking a delicious and nurturing meal for you and your family will be welcomed, and you'll watch fat disappear easily as you gain control of your waistline, and your life.

Here is how I know this:

Do you ever follow advice given to you by strangers on the street?

I doubt it and you shouldn't. It's important for you to understand from where and from whom that advice is coming. While it's true that I am a certified nutritionist, best-selling author, and national speaker, let me tell you a story of who I really am.

When I grew up in a small, blue-collar, Michigan community, I never thought to myself: "I want to be a Transformation Specialist some day." I never thought I would help a single person transform their body, mind or health...let alone impact hundreds of thousands, perhaps millions worldwide.

However, I've accomplished this in a shorter period of time than I thought possible and we're just getting started.

But it didn't start out that way...

When I was younger, I never really thought about anyone but myself, to be completely honest. I chased instant gratification and I figured I had the rest of my life to worry about health.

I'd hit the gym once in a while but my goals were always superficial: Look good for the ladies. I didn't really care what I put into my body as long as it didn't make me sick.

But it was making me sick, from the inside out. I just didn't know it.

I was living in Tampa, Florida during the real estate boom, working in the mortgage industry and although I was making decent money, I was miserable. With stress levels at an all time high from working in a business I hated, and my belly poking out over the top of my jeans, I wondered why I was getting sick four or five times per year.

My mentor at the time pointed out everything in my life that was "out of alignment" and told me I needed to make a major change or be miserable for the rest of my life. And I was only twenty-eight years old at the time.

I wasn't proud of my career, I wasn't proud of my energy levels, I wasn't proud of my body and I felt like I was letting a lot of potential for a better life slip through my fingers.

People who know me know one thing, when I commit to something, I commit "all the way" (I encourage this habit by the way, it's highly effective).

I gave everything away (except my clothes), moved to sunny San Diego and spent a year of my life researching health and learning how to get the body I wanted. Admittedly, I have a bit of an addictive personality as well, so when I started digging into the world of fitness, I wasn't happy to just read books. I wanted to talk to the most prestigious experts who were doing cutting-edge research and getting the best results.

My one criterion, whatever health or fitness regimen I followed was: it would have to be holistically healthy for my mind, body and my soul and NATURAL. No more selling myself short just to try to get a six-pack fast…this was my life we were talking about.

The next year was filled with me weaseling my way in to talk to nationally recognized experts, doctors and fitness specialists. I went to Mexico to a healing center and to places all over California exploring every option I could find.

The results: it all came down to eating good, whole foods, exercising and cultivating a positive mindset. That's the simple explanation, not exactly rocket-science, is it?

I soon realized that the difficult portion would be to re-train myself to enjoy eating good food, working out consistently and staying positive even when the day was trying to beat me down.

But I did it (and you will too).

Along the way, I shared my progress, photos and some very rough Youtube videos on Facebook.com/thinkfeelbecome. I invited my friends to follow my progress. I'm happy to say that the progress went faster than my friends or I ever thought possible.

After only 6 months, I went from 17.2% to 5.75% body fat. And it happened naturally, without drugs, steroids or other unhealthy methods.

Side note: Something very important happens when you enlist others in your success...they join you.

Soon I had my first transformation client who offered me $3,000 to be his virtual coach, from 3,000 miles away and to help lead both him and his wife through the process that I went through. Ninety days later, they both had remarkable results.

Soon, one by one, through word of mouth, people sought me out. My knowledge was growing and with every person I taught, I learned more than they did. I began to understand what limits people, what motivates them and the diverse range of challenges we all face on the way to our health and fitness goals.

Within six months of my first client, I was now being paid $10,000 per client to create the transformation experience for them.

Certain celebrities (whose names must remain private) contacted me for transformation coaching and television producers are now pitching me talk show and infomercial ideas. For a guy who simply shared his success and strategies with those who were willing to listen, the ride has been fun and overwhelming at the same time.

But I keep my focus on my clients. Although each individual faced different challenges, I'm proud to say that 100% of them have not only reached, but often exceeded their fitness goals. That is how I know that what I'm about to teach you works.

7

You don't have to listen to me, but I highly encourage you to open your mind and follow my advice, especially if nothing has worked for you so far.

Chapter 2:

Abs Are Made In The Kitchen

I used to think that doing hundreds of sit ups and long, boring hours of cardio in the gym was the key to a flat stomach and sixpack abs. From crunches, to leg-lifts, to side bends, I did every imaginable exercise for years until I realized that everything was for naught unless I was eating correctly.

Perhaps you experienced the same frustration. If you're like many people, you think that as long as you work out hard, you can probably eat whatever you want. For some people (like athletes) that might be true. For others though, it's a different story. Most people don't have enough hours in the day to work off all of the calories they pour into their body every day.

Furthermore, our bodies respond much better and more quickly to food than they do to exercise. It's been said that 80% of your success is determined by your diet. (I think it's more than that). As important as both of them are, it's the food we put in our body determines the primary shape of our body.

And contrary to popular belief, all calories are not created equal. Fat calories, protein calories, and carbohydrate calories cause our body to react differently. But even more dramatic than that is the

9

difference between whole, nourishing foods (like meats and vegetables) and processed foods (like 90% of the grocery store) in the way our body metabolizes them and uses them for fuel or for fat.

If you drove a sports car, would you put the cheapest gas in it? Some people do.

Recently I was on my way to the beach with my friend Jack. As a passenger in his beautiful BMW M5, which cost more than some people's houses, I was admiring how well it handled and how it really *is* the ultimate driving machine.

We stopped for gas and Jack went into the convenience store to grab a Big Gulp of soda and bag of chips. When he returned he filled up his tank with 93 octane gas. I looked at Jack, then at his Big Gulp, then back at Jack. I asked him, "Why do you put the most expensive gas in your tank, Jack… with gas prices so high?" His answer was exactly what I expected it to be: "Drew, when you own the 'Ultimate Driving Machine' you gotta take care of it— even if it costs a little more."

With a quick glance back at his Big Gulp, I left it at that. Jack never saw his own body as an ultimate anything, let alone the machine that he drives every day of his life. If he did, I'm positive he'd be drinking a bottle of water instead of the chemical soup he calls soda.

Jack is my friend and he doesn't really see himself as having a problem. It's not my job to preach to deaf ears. I find it much more rewarding to help those who have already decided that their lives are worth it, and who believe their bodies are the Ultimate Living Machines.

Train Your Taste To Trim Your Waist

Chapter 3:

Why You Probably Aren't Eating Right . . . Right Now

Junk food tastes good. It tastes like anything *but* "junk." In fact, it's often filling, decadent, comforting, and extremely convenient.

As an expert in health and nutrition, it's shocking to me that many of my clients don't even see it as junk food. They've lived their lives seeing it simply as "food." This is one of the roots of the American obesity epidemic that is my mission to help cure.

That's because this comfort food, which tastes so delicious going in, is also toxic to your health. Junk food is stripped of nutrients, makes you fat, destroys your body's natural healing systems, and creates long-term problems for short-term pleasures.

And this is not news to anyone. Most people *know* they're not eating healthy. So, why do they keep putting this in their bodies?

We could ask my friend Jack. But he'd probably shrug his shoulders and say, "I dunno."

It is not your fault.

13

When is the last time you went the store and bought something labeled "junk food?" Or told the waitress you'd like the "junk food special with a side of empty calories?" That's one reason why it's not your fault; nothing is labeled "Junk Food" (though as you'll see in a minute, if that *were* on the label, it would still likely sell incredibly well).

Instead, there are entire marketing departments with Ivy League MBAs whose sole job is to develop fancy, cute, exciting, and healthy-sounding labels using gimmicks like "healthy choice," "low fat," "sugar-free," and "no trans fats."

They have even hijacked the word "organic" to trick the ill-informed that organic = healthy. Organic cookies may have better ingredients than nonorganic cookies, but they're both loaded with sugar, fat, and calories that will force fat to cling to your body like a bacon-sweater on a hot August night.

Another reason why it's hard to blame you for loving junk food— it's EVERYWHERE and everyone seems to be selling it and/or eating it.

Vegetable farmers don't have massive advertising budgets or executives writing catchy slogans from their boardrooms. As a result, we are bombarded with commercials and billboards for deliciously unhealthy food. It gets in our subconscious. If that kind of food is all that you typically see, it stops being thought of as junk food and starts being thought of as simply "food."

Now, processed food is everywhere and a few generations have grown up with it as normal eating. Thus, convincing someone that Hot Pockets and Happy Meals are junk food is like a stranger telling you that a close friend of yours is a bad person who wishes you harm. But you think, "Gee, he's always been there for me when I needed him and I always have fun when he's around." Would it be easy for you to tell that close friend to take a hike? Probably not.

Lastly, our brains are somewhat wired to think, "If everyone is doing it, then it must not be *that* bad." The processed and fast food industry spends billions of dollars every year to make certain that everyone is doing it—including you.

Of course, when you look at the obesity statistics it also shows that *most* people are overweight, unhappy, and spending billions of dollars to lose weight the "easy way," with dangerous pills, even more dangerous surgeries, and workout gadgets from impulse buys.

So, are you jumping off of the proverbial bridge along with everyone else?

Here is scientific PROOF that it's not your fault

In 1991, the McLean burger was introduced by McDonald's. True to its name, it was leaner than the regular burger. How would you expect a leaner burger to taste? The results might surprise you. According to blind taste tests, many more people preferred the McLean over it's fattier counterpart.

How is this possible? Well you can thank the brilliant scientists at Mickey D's for infusing the burger with artificial fat flavors. Now, a leaner AND better-tasting burger should have been like a better mousetrap. It *should have* been the single best-selling item in McDonald's history. But good luck ordering one today. It was yanked from the menu within one year of its debut due to dismal sales.

This defies logic, but according to a recent University of Texas at Austin research study, one reason for its failure could be as simple as the name itself. "McLean" suggests "McYuck"—not just lower fat and caloric content, but it also implies less tastiness—at least that is according to 60% of Americans.

So is it possible that those who tried the McLean didn't like it because they *expected not to like it*—even though blind taste tests had found it to taste better?

According the to the University of Texas at Austin study titled:

"The Unhealthy = Tasty Intuition and Its Effects on Taste Inferences, Enjoyment, and Choice of Food Products," ...this is exactly what happened. Quoting the study:

> The researchers asked: "What if people consume food that is considered unhealthy, not despite its perceived unhealthiness *but because of it*? That is—what if part of the attractiveness of food lay in its *perceived* unhealthiness?"

> This can happen if consumers intuitively believe that unhealthy food is inherently tastier. The operation of such a belief would increase the chances that people will over-consume food portrayed as less (vs. more) healthy since such food will be expected to taste better.

> Consistent with this idea, the researchers propose that the perceived unhealthiness of food has the ironic effect of enhancing its attractiveness.

> Based on the idea that people assume an inverse relationship between tastiness and healthiness—an assumption that we term the Unhealthy=Tasty intuition—we hypothesize that when information pertaining to assessing the healthiness of food items is provided, foods perceived to be less healthy will be:

> 1. Inferred to taste better

2. Enjoyed more during actual consumption

3. Preferred in a choice task

Scientists being scientists, you just know they were bound to test their theories. And they did.

Results from three controlled experiments confirmed our expectations.

- Participants in Experiment 1 inferred that the less healthy an item, the better its taste.

- Participants in Experiment 2 derived greater actual enjoyment from consuming food that was portrayed as less healthy.

- Finally, participants in Experiment 3 chose an entrée portrayed as more unhealthy when they were prone to seeking enjoyment due to greater hunger.

Interestingly, these results were obtained both among those who agreed and those who *disagreed* that healthiness is inversely related to tastiness.

What use are these results without understanding the reasons *why*?

Let's find out:

According to the researchers, a conjunction of two mechanisms appears to underlie this phenomenon.

1) The hypothesis that unhealthy food is tastier.

2) The hypothesis of "confirmation bias" (a fancy term for the tendency of people to favor information that confirms their beliefs) helps sustain belief in their intuition that unhealthy=tasty.

They also found that the intuition could influence the judgments and decisions of even those who explicitly DISAGREE with the idea that unhealthy food is tastier.

This finding raises the disturbing possibility that consumers may be unaware of *why* they seek and over-consume food that is perceived or portrayed as unhealthy. Without such awareness, controlling one's consumption patterns becomes much more difficult.

So it's really not your fault that you love to eat junk food. But it is your responsibility to train your taste if you want to gain control over how great you look and how energized you feel.

Train Your Taste To Trim Your Waist

Chapter 4:

Your Taste Buds Are Traitors!

Imagine you are sitting in your favorite restaurant, staring down at the menu, deciding which entrée to have for dinner. As you scan the delicious choices, you focus in on the skinless grilled chicken breast with fresh vegetables and a salad. It's directly below the fettuccine Alfredo and above the prime rib with garlic mashed potatoes and bacon mac and cheese.

Notice how you feel inside, how excited are you, when contemplating an order of…the chicken? Does your face grimace a bit? Do you lose all excitement of eating, and feel like your mother has just told you to do your chores?

Compare that with how you feel when you're looking at the chicken fried steak or the pork chops and French fries. Do those feel more inviting?

Now, what if it were possible to flip those feelings around? What if the sight of the seared tuna salad or fresh steamed broccoli made your mouth water in anticipation? What if your taste buds jumped for joy at the thought of eating fresh greens instead of French fries?

Sounds impossible, right? Well if it *were* possible for you, do you think you'd have a much easier time losing that pesky fat around your belly and having a body you'd be proud to display?

My guess is that you wouldn't be reading this book right now. Instead, you'd be shopping for new clothes - the kind that hug your body and help you show off your sexy curves or chiseled physique.

Taste buds are like puppy dogs. If you let them run loose without any guidance, discipline, or restraint, they're going to do whatever they want, making a mess of your body and your life. Soon they'll be uncontrollable and you'll assume you can't teach an old dog new tricks.

They want what they want—just like a two-year-old screaming for a new toy or sugary cereal in the supermarket. Oftentimes they won't quiet down until they get what they want.

But what they want, usually, is not what's healthy for them.

For example, if your child was screaming that they want to play with a book of matches, would you give in and let them play with it? They might not burn the house down, but odds are you'll be standing next to the fire truck asking what went wrong.

Actually visualizing your traitorous and unruly taste buds like this will greatly help you get them under control, and your waistline with too.

22

Now, lets go back to that favorite restaurant where you were looking at the menu. This time, imagine a really fit and healthy-looking couple walk in and sit at a table next to you. She orders the grilled chicken salad and a side of fresh veggies and he orders the salmon and steamed asparagus special. Do you imagine this fit couple grimacing in disgust as they eat their nutrient-dense meal option? Do they seem miserable? It's not that they don't love the taste of your dish; it's that they've tamed their toxic taste buds and trained them to not only enjoy but crave the healthier options. Doing this makes it easy to make the healthy meal choices. That's the cause. The effect is a healthy, sexy body with a lot of energy.

Training your taste buds doesn't happen overnight and it's not always easy, but it is possible for everyone and it can be done much more quickly than you might believe.

Once we recognize the cause and effect, we have little excuse for not following it. At that point, it DOES become your fault if you keep making the same choices over and over.

Train Your Taste To Trim Your Waist

Chapter 5:

How Susan Trained Her Taste Buds

As a transformation specialist who has worked with clients in every imaginable physical shape, I have used the protocol in this book to train the taste buds of my most stubborn clients.

For example, Susan (name changed for anonymity) came to me when every diet, exercise plan, and supplement had failed her. She had been skinny when she was in her early twenties but after having three children and juggling a career and a struggling marriage, she found the pounds piling on as she cooked for convenience and comfort. After two decades of eating the Standard American Diet of processed foods, her taste buds had become toxic. (Is it a coincidence that the acronym for Standard American Diet is S.A.D.?)

Susan had read books on weight loss and had studied what she should eat, but when it came down to making the right menu choice or cooking the healthy option, her willpower disappeared and was replaced by a heavy guilt immediately following her meal. "Next time I'll make a healthy meal," she would tell herself. But the next time never came. "I just can't enjoy eating a plate of veggies or chicken breast, even though I know I should," she told me. "I've eaten the same way since I was a child, so I don't know

25

if I could ever LIKE eating like you do, Drew!" She looked powerless and hopeless as she explained to me that she wished she liked salads, vegetables, and lean meats.

I put her on the protocol that you're about to read in this book and started to train her taste to trim her waist. She took to it immediately because of how gradual the process is and how she can baby-step her way to better health.

On day eight, after losing several pounds, she came to me, and with tears in her eyes said, "Drew, for the first time in my life I'm actually CRAVING vegetables. I can't explain it, but I can feel myself changing." Two weeks later she was regularly cooking and ordering what she is supposed to eat—food that nourishes her from the inside out and melts fat off her hips, thighs, and waist.

She was losing dress sizes, fat, and weight. But she was gaining something even bigger: control. And it wasn't a hard or heavy-disciplined control that forces you to do something you don't want to do. It was like being in charge of her life. Her cravings for sugar, sweets, and fats subsided, and her taste buds welcomed the meals that made her sexy again.

Susan is a brand-new woman with a body she hasn't had since her early twenties. She can still enjoy eating what she used to, but relishes them as a treat on special occasions. She credits this training protocol as the missing link to making her diet work.

Chapter 6:

Old Dogs Mastering New Tricks

Randy (his name changed for anonymity) just turned forty years old when he sought my help. I'll never forget his first email to me.

"Drew, I need your help. I'm a southern-fried redneck from South Carolina and I'm proud of my heritage. What I'm not proud of is what I've done to my body. Turning 40 makes you look at your life, and when I looked in the mirror yesterday I didn't like what looked back at me. My mama is the greatest woman on earth, but I think she spoiled me rotten with her cooking. For years I thought if I'd exercise and go to the gym I could eat whatever I wanted and never gain weight. I was wrong and I need your help.

My problem is that I can't imagine eating what I see you eating in your videos. Juicing vegetables—I mean I'll try anything but I'll be damned if that don't look like a big ol' glass of swamp water. Do deep fried veggies count as healthy? That was a joke. But it's the only part I'm joking about in this email to you. I want your help. I think if I can learn to eat right and like it, I'll have more energy and look a helluva lot better. I got divorced two years ago and haven't had a date since. It's time for a change. Am I hopeless, or can you help me?

27

Yours truly, Randy."

Randy isn't alone. Many of my clients thought they would never be able to actually like the foods they know they should be eating. But every single one of them have witnessed the power of the protocol I'm going to share with you in this book.

Just because you've eaten unhealthy foods your entire life does not mean that you won't grow to love the nutrient-dense and healthy flavors that will transform your body.

Because of their extreme nature, these highly-refined processed foods with their artificial flavors and excessive amounts of sugar, salts, and bad fats literally have burned out your taste buds.

If you're like most people, there are several things that you didn't like at first but you trained yourself to love.

Did you fall instantly in love with your first cup of coffee, beer, wine, or liquor? I didn't. But I wanted the effects they gave me. With coffee, it was all about keeping me awake while pulling all-nighters studying in college. Eventually I learned to love the taste and associated it with meeting friends at cafés or waking up in the morning to a hot cup o' Joe. (I've since switched to a hot cup o' green tea or veggie juice).

It took me years before I liked the taste of beer or could drink liquor without wanting to throw up. But once in college, I was so

28

determined to get the buzz—the *effect* of the alcohol, so I just drank it, taste be damned. Eventually I learned to enjoy the taste of a good microbrew or mixed drink. But I had "trained" my taste to get this result.

Chances are you've done something similar and came to love these things too. Now you have somewhat of an emotional—and part physiological—need for them, right?

It's important for you to know that with time you'll get an even better "buzz" from eating natural, nutritionally dense foods. The constant buzz of strength, energy, emotional balance, and overall health and well-being that comes with fueling our bodies healthfully is real. You can have all of this instead of the temporary physical and emotional highs followed by crashing lows that you get from eating unhealthy processed foods, including over-stimulating substances such as caffeine, alcohol, refined salt, and sugar. The roller coaster of highs and lows that eventually turns primarily into lows will be dead in its tracks.

Train Your Taste To Trim Your Waist

Chapter 7:

How To Train Your Taste To Trim Your Waist

We're about to jump into the protocol now. I'm going to give you simple steps that everyone, at any health or fitness level can follow. You'll notice that most of these steps are mental steps. They may not take much time to do but if you skip them you risk derailing your success. That's why they are so important.

Further, you may be surprised to see how succinct and short this training really is. There is no need for lengthy, overly scientific explanations for every single step in the process. It works. It is based on common sense and scientific principles rooted in natural health methods.

If you choose to continue a scholarly pursuit of the rationale I lay out in this book, I will provide resources for you in the appendix.

Let's train!

<u>Step 1</u>: Decide you actually want to.

Ever heard the phrase "fat and happy?" Some people have no desire to change. But the fact that you're reading this right now means that you DO have that desire. You are taking responsibility

31

for your body, along with your health and happiness, so you have already taken the first step.

Step 2: **Understand that you're not replacing your taste buds, you are training them.**

You'll still enjoy the tastes you always have, but you will crave much healthier alternatives. Just like when training a dog, you're not depriving them from being free and playing once in a while; you're just trying to get them to behave on *your* terms.

Step 3: **Accept that it's a process, not an event.**

Training your taste buds doesn't happen overnight, and sometimes it takes patience and tough love. You should gladly accept the challenge because gaining a victory here is gaining a victory in every part of your life.

Step 4: Define your WHY.

If your reason for wanting to change isn't strong enough, success will be much more challenging. If it's a superficial or weak reason that you're doing this, it's easy to fall back on junk food and abandon the process. However, if you desire to train your taste buds so that you not only *look* better, but also to *feel* better, gain more energy and quality time with your loved ones, improve your confidence and performance at work, and appeal to the opposite sex, then you're one step closer to success.

HOW to define your why

Start off by asking yourself: "What do I want?" When you answer, answer the question exactly...in the positive...meaning "what do I want: to have, to look like, to feel like?"

Resist the temptation to answer what you *don't* want. Too often I'll ask my clients, "What do you want" and they'll say "I want to lose weight, I don't want these love handles, I don't want to feel so tired, I don't want my husband or wife to ignore me."

Do you see the difference? They're answering what they do *not* want. They never get really clear on what they will have or look like when they get what they want. As a result it's harder to get it.

Next, ask yourself, "why is that important" or "what will having that do for me?" Whatever your answer is, keeping asking this question about it until you come to the root.

Example:

Drew: What do you want?

You: I want to have a firm tummy, size 3, with a tight butt. And I want to feel good and energized throughout the day.

Drew: Great...what will having that do for you?

You: Well, it will make me feel good about myself, more confident.

Drew: Great...what will having that do for you?

You: It will make me feel more attractive to my husband, and I know I'll be more attentive as well because I'll feel more confident. And I probably won't complain so much simply because I'm miserable, instead I'll be happier and hopefully sexier to him.

Drew: Great...what will having that do for you?

You: It will help reignite our relationship.

Drew: Great...why is that important to you?

You: Because I love him more than anything and I value our family. If I ever lost it I wouldn't know what to do.

Drew: So your real reason for transforming yourself is to not only look good, but it's to demonstrate to your husband how much you love and value him and your relationship, and by putting your body, mind and spirit first...you feel you'll have more love to give him so you can grow stronger every day of your relationship...is that accurate?

You: Um...yeah.

Drew: Want to eat some donuts right now?

You: (Hopefully shaking your head "no" with a new and steady resolve)

See how easy that is? Try it yourself.

Step 5: The Great Habit Exchange

We learn by repetition and we're creatures of habit. The more often we perform a task in a routine, the more we imprint it on our brains as something natural that we do without thinking. Do you really have to remind yourself to brush your teeth when you wake up, or do you do it as second nature, without thinking?

This is true for our taste buds as well. The healthier we eat and the more healthy choices we make, the less we actually have to think about doing it and the more it becomes second nature.

Habits form quicker than you think. Studies have shown that it takes 21 days of repetitive activity to imprint it as a habit. But you have to do it every day. You have to follow the protocol for those 21 days. If you miss even one day during those 21 you will have to start over from day one.

Don't blame me... blame your brain.

Bad News: You can fall into bad habits in only 21 days as well. Going 21 days without doing something positive is the same thing as doing something negative for 21 days. BAM...habit formed.

Good news. You should be able to do *anything* for 21 days. Especially if the payoff is having a healthy diet and getting the body you've always dreamed of.

So, we're going to focus on a 21-day habit-forming protocol. You'll tell yourself that for the next 21 days, you're going to be disciplined, even if you've never had discipline in your life, and even if you're miserable (which you won't be). But if you do this for 21 days and you feel no different, you're free to go back to your current habits if you wish.

Is It REALLY So Simple a Caveman Can Do It?

That is GEICO's official and trademarked slogan. But I really couldn't think of a better way to explain the next Chapter than to give them credit for what's coming.

Complicated diets and protocols fail. Simple plans succeed.

For the next three weeks—or 21 days—you're going to follow this plan exactly. You're not going to deviate. Although you will likely see some immediate weight loss results, we are more concerned with the mental habits we're forming and initial taste-training results.

I'm about to give you a detailed breakdown of what you're going to eat and what you're going to avoid for the next three weeks. But in general, you're going to be eating simple, boring, but nutritionally packed meals for six out of seven days.

Then one day a week you're going to get to splurge. Not just cheat, but splurge on everything you've been deferring. Notice I didn't say "depriving." More on that below.

36

But I want you to accept the fact that this will at first be boring and sometimes inconvenient. If I sugarcoat it (no pun intended) and tell you that this will be a walk in the park and effortless, then I'd be lying to you, and you deserve to know the truth. And you'd therefore be disappointed and think the plan isn't working, and never trust anything I told you in the future.

Yes, it's way more fun to put the weight on than take it off. The following protocol, however, is specifically designed to make it as painless as possible while creating a long-term, lasting change in your flavor-craving taste buds.

Side note: If you happen to cheat once or twice throughout the week, it doesn't mean you're a bad person, or that you lack willpower, or that you should stop this protocol.

Keep it up the best you can. But know this: I believe in you. Chances are, I don't even know you, but because you're reading this, I believe in you right now, even if you don't believe in yourself.

Doing this 100 percent is easier than doing it 99 percent. Because that 1 percent that you "cheat" will start to eat away at your confidence and at your determination. When you know you gave it 100 percent of your effort, you'll feel so empowered that it makes every choice easier and easier.

I am assuming you're looking for results and *not* academic pontification. I am going to give you some rules and short explanations of why you should follow them. I am not going to dive into the science of how each of these rules work just so you can satisfy scientific curiosity, but there is evidence to support these rules.

These steps are all backed by solid nutritional and scientific principles, but more important, they are proven to work in my clients' lives and others who've put them to use as well. If they make sense to you and you want results, you will follow them to the letter.

Before we jump into this...

I have become one of the leading proponents and spokespeople for the benefits of juicing fresh, organic vegetables and fruits. Many of you may be familiar with my Facebook fan page: Facebook.com/VegetableJuicing

Additionally, my **Juice Up Your Life presentation** at http://www.fitlife.tv/kindle-juiceupyourlife, has helped many people begin their transformation journey

In my opinion, and that of countless scientists and health professionals, there is simply no better nutritional source than a diet rich in live, plant-based foods.

However, I also still eat organic, free range or grass-fed meat, poultry and sustainably fished seafood in moderation, as it fits my metabolic type and makes me feel better. I've tried going raw, vegan and vegetarian, but with the amount of physical activity and weight training I do, my body does not respond as well as when I introduce meat. I've learned to listen very close to my body and I encourage you to do the same.

Ideally and for best results, the next section could and likely should be replaced by going purely vegetarian/vegan for the next 21 days. If you're inclined to do so, I encourage you.

However, most people reading this are looking for a less extreme change and are trying first to flip their habits around. For the sake of the majority, I will use a meat and vegetable-based protocol. Just wanted to clear that up before we begin.

Overview:

Follow this protocol for six out of seven days. For instance, Sunday through Friday, follow this exactly—without deviation. Then choose one day, like Saturday, as your "Cheat and Treat" day. (This will be explained further below)

What did cavemen eat? And why should we care?

The short answer is because we were cavemen (and ate like cavemen) for a lot longer than we've been grocery-cart filling, frozen-dinner-eating, sweet-tooth-satisfying, baked-good-binging, fast-food foragers (a.k.a. "civilized").

Tens of thousands of years ago our ancient ancestors thrived as hunter-gatherers. In fact, scientists estimate that our bodies have been physically modern for over 100,000 years. This means that our genetics really have not dramatically changed since then, even though our bodies have.

The average pre-historic Homo Sapien: muscular, agile, athletic, necessarily strong. If you didn't have these qualities, you were dinner for an animal that did.

The average Homo Sapien today: stressed, flabby, overweight, out of shape, sleep-deprived, unhappy and suffering from many preventable diseases.

What changed? In a word, "agriculture."

In 10,000 BC, give or take a month or so, our species developed the ability to farm. We stayed in one place, formed civilizations and progressed towards our current culture.

Although we developed socially, our bodies never adjusted properly to all the grains that we're now eating. We had tens of thousands, arguably hundreds of thousands of years as hunter-gatherers and only recently we shifted our diet. Unfortunately, our genetics have not shifted with our lifestyle.

Our bodies were used to loading up on meat, vegetables and seasonal fruits. But now we have replaced most of these whole-foods with grains – bread, pasta, corn, rice and the like. Even our trusty government recommends between 6to 11 servings of grains per day.

As a species, we're getting fatter and sicker. Perhaps there are many reasons for this, or perhaps we're fighting Mother Nature too hard and she's fighting back.

Consider this fact: Indians (not Native Americans) discovered how to make crystalline sugar from cane sugar in 350 AD, and for a very long time it wasn't available in most parts of the world. Now it's in nearly everything and we're even manufacturing sugar-like concoctions that are creating even more havoc in our bodies such as high-fructose corn syrup and a host of artificial sweeteners such as saccharin and aspartame.

But you've been told that grains are good for you, right? Grains do have some beneficial properties like fiber and a host of important nutrients. However, they're also composed of carbohydrates,

41

which are turned into glucose, which is a type of sugar. Glucose that is not used for energy during the day is immediately stored as fat.

Most of these issues arise from two substances in grains: lectin and gluten.

Lectins are natural toxins. They give grains the ability to defend themselves against being eaten and consumed by animals or humans. As strange as this sounds, grains have evolved lectins as a defense mechanism. Lectins prevent the gastrointestinal tract from repairing itself from normal wear and tear of digestion. An unhealthy gut can cause more issues than I care to go into.

Gluten is a simple protein. It's found in grains like rye, wheat, and barley. It's very hard on the digestive system. It is water-soluble and creates the elasticity in dough. It also happens to be the primary glue in wallpaper paste. According to researchers, almost one third of the population is sensitive to gluten by showing inflammation in the body.

The resulting inflammation causes a host of conditions such as joint pain, acid reflux, reproductive issues, autoimmune disorders and even dermatitis. Those with a severe reaction are said to have Celiac disease. And just because only one third are considered highly sensitive to gluten does not mean that the other two thirds process it well. They just may not be experiencing the issues in a noticeable manner.

All of these statistics and realizations have recently given rise to a popular dietary trend called the "Paleo Diet" or the "Paleo Lifestyle." However it's not a fad or weird diet. It's simply returning to the way our bodies have been eating for tens of thousands of years, stripping away the processed stuff like unnatural sugars, grains and even dairy.

This means that you'll be eating vegetables, meat (ideally lean) eggs and a small amount of fruit due to the high sugar content of fruit.

Now, it's important that you understand that I'm not going to compare or argue the merits of this diet vs. a completely plant-based or vegan diet, but for the majority of people, this means "eat whole foods" and avoid processed food or foods that cavemen had little-to-no access, like breads or Hot Pockets.

Since it's a plan that includes meat and vegetables, it's much easier for most people (like my transformation clients) to undertake. If you are vegetarian or wish to be, feel free to eliminate meat altogether from the protocol that I'm about to share with you.

Does your menu sound boring? Does it sound impossible to deprive yourself of all the food you're used to eating? Are you nervous you won't be able to do it? I have something up my sleeve that will fix that in a second. Stick with me.

Side Note: The "Paleo Diet" has a lot of avid fans and adherents right now. It should be noted that this book is NOT a complete or dogmatic "how to" on everything "Paleo." You may find minor alterations in my protocol and abbreviated descriptions. This book is not indoctrination to one diet or another; it's a protocol that's been proven to work by my personal clients. For your benefit, at the end of this book I will give you more resources to read from experts in the Paleo Lifestyle.

Rule 1: White Is Not Right

Most white foods are not naturally white. Bread, rice, or anything with flour that is white has been bleached white using chemicals and processes to strip away not only the color, but the nutrients that are vital for your nutrition. White, processed foods are basically empty calories, and you may as well be consuming spoonfuls of sugar.

Unfortunately, you'd be amazed at how many foods fall into this category. This will seem like the hardest rule, but it will have the greatest impact on your waistline and your health.

So avoid white carbohydrates or food that can be easily turned white.

Avoid: All bread, all rice, cereals, tortillas, pastas, noodles, potatoes, anything fried in breading, or anything made with flour.

Rule 2: Don't Do Dairy

There are a number of reasons why dairy does NOT do a body good, despite the billion-dollar advertising claim to the contrary. There is ample evidence that the over-consumption of dairy products creates all types of unwanted effects, including sugars that your body does not need and hormones fed to the cows to speed up their production that can cause havoc in our bodies. Disregard all of that for a moment.

I'll just leave you with one of my observations about dairy products:

Milk is a wonder of nature. It's evolved to be a perfect food source for the offspring of all mammals, channeled from the body of the mother into her offspring. It has the needed enzymes, fats, and proteins to allow this offspring to survive. Each animal produces a chemically different form of milk for its young. Each animal's milk is evolutionarily optimized for that species, including human breast milk.

All animals eventually and naturally wean themselves off of this nutritional source at a young age when their bodies are ready for whole foods.

Humans are the only animal that continually drinks milk (or eats milk products) throughout adulthood. And we're the only species that drinks the milk of another species while we're doing it.

If we are going to drink milk, it makes more logical sense that we'd buy human breast milk at the store and use that in our cereal, doesn't it? But that's just gross. We would never do that.

That's just something to get your hamster wheel spinning.

But the bottom line is that if you want to transform your body and your health; if you want to train your taste to trim your waist, follow this guideline and it will be a much faster and easier path.

Rule 3: Drinking Donuts

How do you drink a donut? Simply keep drinking soda pop and store bought fruit juices and all of the sugar-loaded drinks that so many Americans are used to gulping down. They may as well be donuts.

This rule was originally called "Drinking Don'ts"…like "Don't drink soda!"

But "Don'ts" looks enough like "Donuts" and the epiphany occurred. So now, every time you reach for that soft drink, think of yourself as literally gulping down a donut.

Diet drinks with artificial sweetener count as donuts as well. Not for the sugar content but because they're highly processed and arguably very toxic to your system. Additionally, we're training your taste buds not to crave sugar here.

So what can you drink? Drink as much water, unsweetened iced tea or hot tea that you can. Fresh squeezed vegetable juice (for this protocol, fruit juice has too much sugar, stay away from that, including orange juice).

You may have a moderate amount of coffee if you wish, as long as it's black and unsweetened. For many of you, that will keep you from drinking coffee altogether as well.

Contrary to popular belief, you actually CAN live off water as your only beverage in life.

And of course I wouldn't end this rule without addressing alcohol. Alcohol is a sugar. We're deferring and avoiding sugar on this plan. This may be even harder for you to give up than breads, but if you want results you will do it. At least for the time you're training your taste.

Free Reader Bonus

Only Available To You

As A Thank You For Reading

"Train Your Taste To Trim Your Waist."

Visit http://trainyourtaste.com/reader-bonus

Your Six-Day Weekly Meal Plan for the Next Three Weeks

I'm going to make this easy and list the number of foods you are free to eat. This is not an exhaustive list but a list of the most common foods you can consume. Feel free to mix and match and get creative. But remember, whole foods only.

Also, in my daily diet I try to choose only organic, sustainably and responsibly farmed meats and vegetables and I encourage the same from you. However, for some people, cost and availability are an issue. Organic and natural is best, but buying conventional meats and produce while giving up processed food is definitely a good start and better than nothing.

So, cutting out processed foods, you are left with only those that occur naturally.

Proteins

- Chicken: Look for organic or free-range when available
- Turkey
- Beef: Grass-fed, not grain-fed as grain can cause the same issues in animals as humans.
- Fish/sea food: wild-caught is better due to toxins that can occur in farmed fish.
- Pork
- Organic eggs including yolk

Nuts*

- Almonds
- Pecans
- Brazil nuts

*Caution about nuts. Most people eat 10x the amount of nuts they should because they are seeking the crunchy texture. Nuts are full of good fats, but they're full of fat nonetheless. The rule is, no more than a small handful at a time (if you're trying to trim your waist).

Vegetables

ALL of them, as much as you want. For example: broccoli, cauliflower, asparagus, beets, salad greens, cabbage, squash, bell peppers, spinach, kale, lettuce, carrots (in moderation, due to sugar content), etc.

Oils

Limit oils reasonably, but stick to olive oil, coconut oil and avocado oil when possible.

What About Restaurants: Temptation Central?

While you are training your taste, I encourage you to make as many meals for yourself, at home as possible. This is the easiest way to stick to the program. But I know that's not feasible for everyone so I will give you some alternatives.

It might be challenging at first but you can typically find something in the above categories at almost any restaurant. Even if they charge more to substitute for the healthy options, pay it. It's well worth the additional money. Think of it as a six-pack tax. If the grilled chicken breast comes with rice and beans, but you can substitute that for fresh steamed vegetables for an extra two dollars, isn't your waistline worth the money?

The bad news is that most restaurants are tailored for people eating the Standard American Diet and are going to be overloaded with unhealthy options. It may appear that there are no healthy choices on the menu, or at least no healthy choices that look the least bit appetizing to you.

Here is where I like to turn the process into a game of Menu Hide-N-Seek. I challenge myself to find the healthiest options on any menu and make any necessary combinations to do so. I know what I will and will not eat, so it becomes a Sherlock Holmes style game of process-of-elimination.

When I find the meal that will nourish my body and help me achieve my goals, I feel as though I have won. I have beaten the establishment. I have conquered the menu. This makes me feel stronger because I turned it into a challenge. You can (and should) do this too.

Another trick I use in restaurants when looking at the menu, being seduced by all of the flavorful but unhealthy options, is to ask this question of each option: "will eating this option get me closer to or further away from my goal?" Usually that's all it takes to make the right decision.

One last thought on restaurants: some styles of them have healthier choices than others. Traditionally, Italian restaurants are loaded with pasta, pizza, breadsticks and all other types of tempting flavors. It can be challenging to find something that fits in your meal plan here. If you can find the grilled chicken or other meats and pair it with a salad or vegetables, do it. But I encourage avoiding Italian restaurants due to the temptation factor.

Do you love Mexican food? Good news. You have options. Skip the tortilla chips and order the chicken or steak fajitas with fresh vegetables, or indulge in a big salad and use salsa as your dressing instead of ranch.

Vegetarian fajitas are a wonderful alternative as well especially if you're trying to limit the amount of meat you eat, which I encourage.

This brings me to a point I must address about most restaurant meats. In my own diet I stick to about 80% vegetables and whole foods. I love eating a raw, plant-based diet most of the time. I do eat organic, pasture-raised or grass-fed beef. I am very concerned about the treatment of the animals, as well as the hormones that go into most commercially produced meat.

For these reasons, I personally skip most restaurant meat dishes unless they fall into my criteria above, which is rare. But these suggestions are assuming that you are not yet as concerned with these factors and are primarily looking for a transition to a better nutritional lifestyle without going through extreme changes that could derail your progress.

If you *are* conscious and concerned with eating only organically (which I recommend) or ethically opposed to eating meat, then I highly encourage you to follow those convictions and take this program even further. Your body will thank you for it.

Rule 4: Eat five to six smaller meals per day.

Surprisingly, it's often more challenging for my clients to increase the frequency of their meals rather than the consistency. By cutting portion size in half and doubling the number of times you eat per day, you remind your metabolism never to go into fat-storing mode. This is one of the biggest tricks of fast weight loss when combined with healthy meals. Simply eat a smaller meal every three to four hours.

The inconvenience factor, combined with the fact that most people don't think about food except for three times per day, throws many off track. One simple trick is to program the reminder or alarm on your phone to go off every three to four hours, reminding you to eat something. Remember, we're going for the habit here.

Example Meals

Breakfast: Choose one per day.

A. One to three eggs, sweet potato hash browns, broccoli or cauliflower, ¼ avocado.

B. Coconut milk (¼–½ cup), berries (raspberries, blueberries, strawberries, or blackberries), and nuts (almonds, walnuts, or macadamia).

C. One-to-three-egg omelet with veggies (peppers, onions, mushrooms), ¼ avocado, add salsa if you'd like.

Lunch: Choose one per day.

A. 4–6 oz salmon over mixed greens salad topped with nuts (almonds, walnuts, macadamia nuts, etc.). *add additional vegetables like beets, sweet potato, apple, etc. if this isn't enough substance.

B. 4–6 oz ground beef, vegetable of choice (broccoli, asparagus, cauliflower, etc.) ¼ avocado or a handful of olives.

C. ½ –1 cup tuna salad (1 can tuna, ¼ onion, 1 tbsp olive oil, salt & pepper) with a side of cooked carrots and a vegetable of your choice.

Dinner: Choose one per day.

A. Ground turkey burger, steamed broccoli and asparagus, ¼ avocado or coconut flakes.

B. ¼–½ lbs. shrimp, kale or spinach salad with nuts or olives, sliced apples, onions, and balsamic vinegar.

C. Large mixed greens salad with grilled chicken and veggies topped with balsamic vinaigrette.

Snacks: Choose one per snack time.

A. ¼ avocado with sea salt

B. 2-3 oz. protein of your choice

C. 1 oz. Coconut Flakes or nuts

D. D. 1-3 oz. Plain Beef or turkey jerky (Often jerky is flavored with teriyaki or other seasonings that are loaded with sugar. It's best to avoid the sugary flavored jerky in favor of the plain or original flavor.)

These are merely example meals. The point is to pick from the food list above and combine them. Try to eat smaller quantities of food but eat more often. However, do not count calories or portion sizes too much. We are trying to keep the training regimen simple enough for you to stick to it.

SUCCESS TIP: Write down your cravings in a journal or in a notepad of your smart phone. Anytime you are craving lasagna or pie or a sandwich, write down in explicit detail exactly what you want. This will not only help satisfy the appetite for it (don't ask me how, it just works) but it will help for the next rule...

Rule 5: Your One-Day-Deferred Binge . . . I mean "Treat" Day

This will feel really weird and wonderful at the exact same time. There will be a part of you that even feels a bit naughty for indulging while the other part of you will welcome it with open arms.

One day per week, fulfill all the week's cravings in one day, or even in one meal (for those more disciplined). Today is no-holds-barred. You can eat everything and anything on the "do not eat list." In fact, feel free to make yourself a little sick today.

Why? Won't I ruin all my progress? The answer is no. In fact you'll probably accelerate fat loss for the reasons I explain below.

First, the psychological reason we're doing this is because it makes it much easier to get through the week of eating healthy. You go from depriving to deferring. If you think that you'll never be able to eat cheesecake again, you'll miss it badly. If you know you only have to wait a few more days to indulge, you'll see the light at the end of the tunnel and find the willpower you need to keep pressing on with this protocol.

The second, more fun and astounding reason is that research and empirical evidence shows that doing this actually accelerates fat loss.

Our metabolism tends to protect us from starvation (thanks Caveman) by slowing down when it senses a caloric deficit, and therefore burning less fat for fuel. This scheduled "treat and cheat" day reminds your metabolism to get back to work. In fact, the caloric overload causes it to work overtime, quickly burning what you just dumped into your body. When you resume your nutritional overload and caloric deficit the following day, your metabolism is still working hard, only this time it's stripping off the fat from around your waist.

Here's the other reason this method works. You will feel so good all week from your new eating habits, no bloating, more energy, less lethargy and then THIS day will cause massive disruption that shows you how bad you'll feel when you eat like this. It will taste good but actually make you crave veggies and lean meats.

Earlier I mentioned the benefits of creating a craving-journal. I've included a basic one here that you could easily recreate in your own journal or on your computer.

Treat Day Craving Journal

Use this worksheet to keep track of your weekly cravings, the ones you are *deferring* until your chosen treat day. If you're craving pancakes on Wednesday. Write them down in the breakfast section here. Fried chicken? Stick it in the lunch section. Go crazy. Today is not about healthy choices. It's a short-term mental exercise designed for specific results.

The act of writing it down has a somewhat magical effect of transferring the desire from your mind to the paper. And for many people, it quells the intensity of the craving by reminding you that you're not "going without" but "going *until.*"

Rules for the Day: There are no rules. Eat everything you've been deferring.

For Breakfast I will eat:

- _____
- _____
- _____

For Lunch I will eat:

- _____
- _____
- _____

For Dinner I will eat:

- _____
- _____
- _____

Are you nervous about derailing your discipline from the week? Don't be. Many people report greater weight loss from this due to the metabolic activity spike. Further, this has the strange effect of showing you how poorly your body feels after indulging versus how good you have likely felt during the week.

Rule 6: **Face yourself in the mirror each day and remind yourself…**

…That you're doing this for your health, your life, and your family. You're giving your taste buds the same tough love you'd give a child or a pet when you're trying to steer their behavior toward more positive choices. Then remind yourself you can do anything for twenty-one days and that the results will be worth it, because *you* are worth it.

Rule 7: **Forgive yourself**

This rule may be one of the most important which is why I left it until last. Few acts are as powerful as forgiveness and we're going to start with the person in the mirror.

You will forgive yourself for whatever actions have brought you to the point in your life where you're not happy with the way you look or feel. You've taken responsibility for the actions that have gotten you here, you have owned the actions and realized that everything is a matter of cause and effect.

Now it's time to forgive yourself for those past actions (or inactions) which have not served your best interest. Forgive yourself for any ignorance you had of the right way to eat and then commit to make a positive change moving forward.

61

You also need to prepare to forgive yourself in case you find yourself stumbling with this new taste-training regimen.

I want you to follow it to the letter. I want you to be so disciplined that you complete every step easily. I believe that you will. I also recognize that some will have greater challenges than others.

Without giving you a green light to cheat on the program, I want you to know that if you do cheat, if you stumble or falter, it's ok. Keep going. Do not get so upset with yourself that you stop the program. Push on.

If you succumb to temptation, if you cheat on the program, don't quit the program. Instead, notice the way that guilt feels and use it to fuel yourself the next time you're tempted to get off track. Realize you are only cheating yourself and that you can forgive yourself and continue on the path.

The simple fact that you're making the choice to do is a victory for you. Now it's time to see yourself through to the end, which I believe you will do!

Chapter 8:

Day 22

Congratulations! You've done what few others will. It's likely you'll have developed a new and healthy habit that will make it easier to make the right meal choice.

But your journey is just beginning. You will still occasionally crave foods that aren't healthy for you. Temptation will still be lurking. You didn't transform your taste buds, you've simply trained them and shown them that you are the boss.

One of the main victories is that you'll know you can do it. Small steps lead to big gains.

Diet and willpower often fail because we set too high of goals too quickly. We tell ourselves we want six-pack abs and will stop at nothing until we get them. Then we bust our butt for two to three months and if they haven't shown up, we get frustrated and quit. You can still have that goal, but if you're starting from square one, you need some smaller goals and victories to celebrate. The 21 day habit exchange is exactly that.

So what's next?

If you've made it this far, are happy with yourself and motivated to keep going, I'm going to introduce you to a very specific protocol that is responsible for amazing changes and true transformations, not only in the way you look, but how you feel and how you think.

It might sound extreme, it might sound impossible and it might sound crazy. But if you open your mind and follow along the next few pages I will guarantee it is one of the single healthiest things you could ever do.

Introducing the Alpha Reset.

The Alpha Reset is a five-day super nutrient infusion protocol that simultaneously cleans out your system, detoxifies your taste buds, and floods your body with the nourishment it craves.

Of all the health protocols that my clients undergo, this one has the greatest effect but also the greatest initial resistance. Many people are intimidated or think there is no way they could complete it, and when they do, they wonder why they never did it before.

The term "fast" brings up unpleasant images for some people. The most frightened of them believe they'll face excruciating hunger pains all day long. Meanwhile, others think they're starving their body and that it's not healthy to avoid food for several days. Many have heard that this is what anorexics do to lose weight and it must be unhealthy.

Both of these scenarios and arguments are completely devoid of reality. In fact, for most people, a correctly performed fast gives the body incredible benefits.

In this case, we will be "juice fasting."

And although we're starting this with a juice *fast*...it will likely become a major part of your everyday lifestyle as you feel and see the benefits it has on your body.

Don't run away from me now, this is where the fun and success really begin.

Understanding the Juice Fast

You've probably heard of juice fasts. You may even have tried one more than once as a way to lose weight quickly. But a juice-fast is much more than a means of dropping a few pounds. A juice fast is a way to cleanse your body and prepare it for your continued transformation.

First, what is "Juicing" and how is it different or better than blending or smoothies?

For what it's worth, since fruits have so much sugar (even natural sugar is sugar) I usually recommend a majority of your juices and smoothies be primarily veggie based.

Let's begin with blending smoothies as most people are familiar with the concept or have a blender at home. Blenders blend the juice and pulp and fiber together to create a drinkable form of mixed fruits and vegetables.

A juicer on the other hand is a machine that squeezes only the juice, the life blood of the vegetable, where all the vitamins and antioxidants are stored and separates them completely. Then you drink the juice.

"But isn't fiber good for me?" You say.

It is good for you. And I love fresh smoothies. They're more filling and keep your digestive tract working to break down the remainder of the fiber and pulp while getting the juice too. This is good for your metabolism and the filling effect keeps you from eating food to satiate your hunger.

But the first benefit to juicing is that you can ingest more juice when the pulp is removed, thus more vitamins and nutrients can nourish your body, which is likely starving for them. The second benefit to juicing is that your body doesn't have to work so hard to break down the fiber, thus getting to enjoy the benefits immediately.

When you think about your body, it's really like a big human juicer anyway. The fruit and veggies go in, the body extracts the juice and expels the stuff it can't use. You're just giving your body a break and doing some of the work for it.

Later, I'll give you a great resource on picking a juicer if you don't already own one.

So how does Juice Fasting work?

Unlike trendy quick-fix diets, a juice fast nourishes *and* cleanses your body at the same time. It shakes your system free of toxins and revitalizes your energy levels. Think of it as a reboot of your entire body and soul. A pure juice regimen, maintained for one to three days, gives your body the simple nutrition it needs in a pure, organic package. And focusing your nutrition in this way for a few days will also allow you to center your mind. By paring down your food choices and freeing your body from the energy that it takes to process your typical diet, you'll be able to reconnect body and spirit, and sense which parts of your body need extra attention.

A juice fast is meditation for your body.

The visualization techniques you use each day help you to zero in on your goals. They fuel your transformation and keep you on target. A juice fast does the same thing. Lots of people focus on their body in a superficial way, mostly being concerned only with how it looks. People neglect to really listen to what their body is trying to tell them.

A juice fast helps to identify those subtle cues that the body is sending out. How do you feel? Do parts of your body feel tired? Do other parts feel more energized? Nature has built in a sophisticated defense system. Your body feels tired when it needs nutrients. You feel pain when something is not working properly.

You need to learn to pay attention to your *physical* thought processes as much as you do your mental and spiritual ones. All of the processes are in this together.

What do I need?

The first thing you need for a juice fast is a willingness to make a dynamic change. The next thing is, well, juice.

We can't use a blender for this because it leaves the pulp in juice. And as much as I love a smoothie and the benefits of fiber, it's not part of the Alpha Reset. We are giving your digestive tract a break from breaking it all down.

So you need a juicer that squeezes the live juice out of the vegetables and discards the pulp. But how do you know which juicer to buy?

There are many models on the market and they range in price from $50 for a juicer that will likely burn out in a month to over $1,000 for the really high-end models.

But I recommend you find a juicer somewhere in the middle.

Let's start juicing!

Ready to begin? All you need are some fresh, locally-sourced organic fruit and vegetables, water, and a juice extractor. With a juicer, you end up with juice—the fresh, pure, natural heart of the plant. It is important to use organic fruits and vegetables, not only because they contain more nutrients, but also because they are pesticide-free. The point of a juice fast is to get rid of toxins, not to add a few more to the mix.

What can I juice?

What you juice is up to you, but you typically don't want to combine more than three fruits or vegetables together. As a rule of thumb, especially when just starting out, I'd stick to one category at a time— fruit or vegetable.

The two don't always play well together in a glass. Also, fruit can spike your blood sugar levels and could cause your energy to crash later on in the day. Personally the two fruits I go with if I absolutely need them are pears and apples, they tend to be a little bit lower in sugar (and of course lemons). But feel free to mix and match, come up with your own juice recipes, and be sure to share any amazing new blends you develop with us at Facebook.com/vegetablejuicing.

To make things easy, I've broken fruits and veggies down into six categories. They'll help you better understand what each fruit or vegetable type does for your body, as well as help you keep your nutrition balanced.

While you're on the juice fast, you'll also need to drink at least six glasses of room temperature water each day. Your body processes room temperature water more effectively, because it doesn't have to work so hard to warm it up. When you drink ice water your body has to go into over-drive to metabolize it and anything else in your stomach. And, to keep yourself fully energized, drink a juice mix every 90 minutes or whenever you feel like you are hungry.

Six to Mix

Fruits and vegetables fall into six basic groups. Generally, the fruits and vegetables in these categories mix well. But once you get the hang of juicing, you may want to try some more daring cross-category mixes. I've included a few examples here to get you started. But, again, it's up to you. Juicing is fun! Try things out and then share what you like.

1.   Acidic Fruits: Oranges, grapefruits, pineapples, lemons, and limes. These fruit juices are high in water and sugar, as well as Vitamin C. They will flush your system, but not keep your energy high.

2.   Vegetable Fruits: Tomatoes and cucumbers. Tomatoes also have high acidity, but paired with cucumbers they have a cooling effect. Vegetable fruits don't have the energy punch of leafy or root vegetables, but they're great for a medium-energy burn that nourishes your mind and body.

3.   Leafy Greens: Lettuce, cabbage, spinach, parsley, and watercress. Leafy greens are densely packed with vitamins and minerals. They release energy more slowly and keep you nourished for a longer period of time.

4.   Root Veggies: Beets, carrots, onions, and radishes. Root veggies are the jewel of slow-burn energy. Some people like to add ginger to this category, and that's fine if you like a little fire in your juice. They sustain physical energy while providing mental energy. There's no quick boost here, but you have a time-release nutrient blast that will last you for hours.

5.   Sweet Fruits: Prunes and grapes. These fall into the same category with acidic fruits. They flush the system and give you a natural fructose burst. Don't count on them for hours of energy. Acidic fruit and sweet fruit juices should be followed up with one of the slower burn categories. Try a leafy-green or root-veggie juice as a follow-up to a day started with acidic fruits.

6.   Sub-Acid Fruits: Apples, pears, peaches, plums, apricots, cherries, lemons and limes as well as berries. These tasty fruits

have the high impact boost of acidic and sweet fruits paired with a slower energy-release. They're great for the middle of the day when you're feeling some lag.

Finer Points:

Different people enjoy different tastes. Some like it hot, and some, well, don't. If you find that your juice is a little bitter, try adding lemon and lime. A dash of apple cider vinegar will cool down vegetables that are too spicy, and a bit of ground ginger root will perk up a juice mix that is too bland.

If this is your first juice fast, you might want to focus on the most easily digestible leafy greens and vegetables, and approach the acids and root vegetables more sparingly. As you become more comfortable with occasional juice fasts, you'll be mixing like a pro and coming up with your own juices. Throwing some seasonal herbs into the mix is another great way to make your juice fast more delicious. Again, you know what you like, so if you're not a fan of the bitter, you might want to avoid cilantro, and if you have problems with acid reflux, keep away from high acidic mixes.

Another great tip for newbie juicers is to be colorful in your choices. Don't stick with one fruit or vegetable color. Make sure that you vary the color mix throughout the day. The colors of fruits and vegetables give you clues about their nutritional value.

As a quick guide:

72

<u>Red/Orange</u>: These fruits and veggies are generally high in Vitamin C, Vitamin A, potassium, and antioxidants. Think tomatoes and strawberries.

<u>Yellow/Orange</u>: Loaded with Vitamin C, Vitamin A, and potassium, these fruits/veggies can boost your immune system and improve vision. Think carrots, peaches, and pineapples.

<u>White/Yellow</u>: Good for the heart, these veggies and fruits also help control cholesterol. Think bananas, mushrooms, and onions. I wouldn't recommend juicing bananas or mushrooms though.

<u>Green</u>: Dark greens pack a power punch of potassium and Vitamin K. They help strengthen bones and teeth, improve vision, and contain fiber. Think kale, spinach, and bok choy.

<u>Blue/Purple</u>: These dark dynamos boost urinary tract health and memory function, slow aging, and taste great. Think cranberries, blueberries, egg plant, and purple grapes as well as my personal favorite: the mighty beet.

A juice fast is an amazing way to get in touch with your body, but you can't live on juice alone. Many of my transformation students go through what is called an Alpha Reset which is a 5 day fast. As you come off a juice fast, you'll have to reintroduce your body to eating. Start simple with things like brown rice or quinoa, easy-to-digest vegetables and fruits and lots of water. In a few days, your body will be more than ready to resume the nutritional routine that you've come to embrace, but there's a lot to be learned from juicing.

Write it down!

It's a great idea to keep a special juicing journal during your juice fasts. You may want to re-read it before each fast. It will give you a great overview of your journey and help you hear what your body is trying to say. Take special note of how you feel when and after you juice.

Don't stop juicing!

I like to juice fast seasonally. Not only is this a great way to tune yourself to the changes of the year, but at the beginning of each season, you'll be able to find the most delicious fruits and vegetables at your local farmer's market. You might even want to consider signing up for a CSA (Community Supported Agriculture) or at least subscribing to their emails or liking their Facebook page, so you can check out seasonal recipes. You often find some great juicing ideas there. You might even want to share a few recipes of your own.

And even after your juice fast is over, you can still enjoy the amazing recipes you've found and develop a few new ones. Juices mix perfectly into your everyday nutritional routine. People have been distilling fruits and vegetables down to their essential minerals and nutrients for years, and there's a reason why: they're delicious!

Here are four of my favorite vegetable juices so you can see what goes in them.

If you're new to juicing, it's perfectly natural for these to appear unappetizing, even gross or disgusting. A small part of me hopes these recipes appear that way to you now. That is because once you taste them, the surprised and delighted look on your face will be priceless (I just wish I were there in your kitchen to see it for myself).

The Green Energizer

This drink is one of my favorite weight-loss juices.

- 2 apples
- 1 cucumber
- 1 lemon (peeled)
- 1 cup of kale
- 3 stalks of celery
- 1/4 bulb of fennel
- 1-inch piece of ginger
- 1/4 head of romaine lettuce

Kale is high in beta-carotene. Kale also has a significant supply of vegetable protein that is amazing for your body. Next time you are at the market, look for kale's healthy but ignored cousins—Swiss chard, mustard greens, and collards.

MEGA GREEN MAN (a.k.a. THE DAY SLAYER)

If you are in an energy slump, this is the juice for you, getting you revved up and ready to slay the day.

- 2 carrots
- 1 broccoli floret
- 2 collard green leaves
- 1 ginger knuckle
- 2 handfuls of spinach
- 1 handful of dandelion greens
- 1/4 beet
- 1 lemon

This juice is one of my personal favorites. Trim up the carrots so they fit in the juicer. If the lemon is not organic, trim the skin off that as well. Wash the rest of the vegetables with "veggie wash" and get ready to dominate life.

The Body Purifier

I drink this juice to flush out the necessary toxins and give my heart a boost.

- 2 carrots
- 1 cucumber
- 1/2 cauliflower
- 1/2 of a beet

Cut the top off the carrots and peel the skin off of the cucumber if it is not organic. Many times, if the beet is not organic, the chemicals will be at the base where the beet and the stems connect. Make sure it is clean or cut it off completely.

Life Regenerator Blood Boost

Drink this juice to purify and give your blood the iron it needs. A 180g serving of spinach (boiled) contains 6.44 mg of iron, whereas one 170g hamburger patty has at most 4.42 mg.

- 5 carrots
- 1 handful of parsley
- 2 radishes
- 6 spinach leaves
- 4 lettuce leaves
- 1 piece of ginger

77

Trim the tops of the carrots off and wash all your vegetables. Put them in the juicer and enjoy. Drink this juice slowly. I usually spend 15 minutes drinking a juice like this. You've heard the saying, "chew your juice."

And before we continue on to the next Chapter, if you are ready to try juicing and want my **best selling book on Amazon**, simply click the link below or visit…

Juicing Recipes For Vitality And Health

By Drew Canole on Amazon

https://www.amazon.com/dp/B007DDQYCU

Chapter 9:

Let's Recap The Protocol

1. Decide you actually want to train your taste, then...

2. Understand you're not replacing your taste buds, your training them

3. Accept that it's a process not an event

4. Define your "why"

5. Commit to the 21 Day "Great Habit Exchange"

   -White is not right

   -Don't do dairy

   -Drinking Donuts

   -Meal Plan: Lean meat, vegetables, eggs, nuts 6 days per week

   -Deferred Binge (aka Cheat & Treat): One day or one meal per week

   -Alpha Reset Juice Fast for 3 to 5 days.

Simple isn't it? Taken in chunks like this you can see just how do-able this really is.

What comes next?

Get your Reader Bonus at

TrainYourTaste.com/reader-bonus

Chapter 10:

(((The Ripple Effect)))

"A victory here is a victory everywhere!"

By now you've read the protocol I use for my transformation clients to give them an advantage over most people who start off with good intentions to change their eating habits, go on a diet or try to lose fat. And this is one of many reasons that the people who train their taste first, achieve a much higher success rate than those who try to wing it on willpower alone.

You'll probably notice that even though you may be tempted to eat the food you shouldn't the next time you sit down at a restaurant, your training takes over and you smile as you enjoy the option that nourishes your body, not just your taste buds.

By focusing on this small but important challenge it makes every aspect easier. When you love the food that loves you back, eating nourishing foods becomes second nature. The foods transforms your body, gives you more energy, focus and determination to keep it up.

My clients report that their relationships improve, job performance increases and their attitude becomes much more positive.

This is where the transformation process begins. And transformation is a never-ending journey with ups and downs along the way.

I'm not saying it will be easy though, I'm saying it will be worth it.

What does the Transformation Process really look like?

You have gone through part of it already as it pertains to transforming your taste buds to enjoy healthy foods. This was a small but focused commitment. Amplifying this commitment becomes much easier once you have already achieved victory. To truly transform you need to take the process to every level of your life.

Earlier in the book we discussed defining your "Why." We surpassed the superficial reasons for change and we made the reasons much more integrated into your entire life.

The next step is to re-define what I call your "Why-Dentity."

Knowing *why* you are doing something is half the battle. Knowing who you really are is the other half. Your identity is who you see yourself as, whether it's a fat person longing to be skinny or a fit, healthy person trapped inside a temporarily unfit body, you must get clear on that. Your answer to that question determines most of your success, or lack thereof.

Your identity determines how you behave in every situation, even when nobody is looking. Especially when nobody is looking. This is why it's much easier to make those choices when you truly see yourself as a fit, healthy, vibrant person who may be temporarily in another situation.

This is redefining your Why-Dentity (and the subject of one of my next books).

The next step in transformation is often overlooked but equally important: Enlisting the support of your family and friends.

Without a support team in place to root you on, help you out and encourage you, making the right choices is exponentially more difficult. Unfortunately many people have friends and family who consciously or unconsciously sabotage and work against their progress. They ridicule and minimalize the efforts of the person trying to transform because seeing it happen makes them uncomfortable.

It's hard to measure, but this may be the root cause of once dedicated people falling off the wagon and abandoning their dreams of transformation. It is the reason that I take such special care to ensure that those whom I oversee their transformation, have the tools and resources to enlist their support team at home. And it's the reason I foster that same feeling between all of my transformation clientele with each other.

After these two primary milestones have been achieved, the remainder of the transformation process happens much easier and more quickly.

From exchanging bad habits for good ones and getting educated on the right choices and why to make them, the person's Why-Dentity takes over and never fails to surprise me at how much they achieve in such a short period of time.

Proper nutrition and exercise are the components that create the most lasting change and with so much conflicting information it's important to choose the programs that are right for your body and metabolic type.

It's also important to go into a transformation with the mindset that once transformed, you will help others achieve what you have. Even if the only thing you do is inspire others as to what's possible, keeping this frame of mind causes you to learn and integrate what you have been taught at a much deeper level.

When you go into the process with the eventual goal of helping others, it's like you carry more responsibility, it makes you less likely to falter because you know that others are depending on you. Pretty powerful, is it not?

This is where the "ripple effect" really comes in.

It's not just about what training you taste does for you. It's what your success and actions eventually do for others. One-by-one we can heal the world. When you believe that, as I do, it gives you immeasurable strength.

I know this because I've seen it happen. I receive photos of remarkable transformations from people who've done it and then thanked me for providing information, entertainment and inspiration.

Some of them are my personal transformation clients. Some of them are my friends. Others I may never have met personally... but they make me believe that anyone can transform their life when they know why they want to do it and have the information about how to do it.

None of us succeed alone. We all have someone getting our back, believing in us and picking us up when we feel we can't do it.

That's why my motto is:

"Remember, we're in this together."

I encourage you to join me and the community that I affectionately call "Fit Lifers."

We realize that our choices create the bodies we live in and the life that follows. We accept responsibility for our current condition, acknowledge our failures and then make the right choices to take glory in our success. Most people will never feel as good as we feel or look as good as we do because they haven't decided that they're worth it.

Have you decided that you're worth it yet?

Claim your Free Bonus a Thank You for Reading

"Train Your Taste To Trim Your Waist."

http://www.trainyourtaste.com/reader-bonus

RESOURCES

How to stay in touch with Drew Canole

- Website: Fitlife.tv

- Twitter.com/Drewcan777

- Youtube.com/fitlifetv

Also Get Drew Canole's Best-Selling Amazon Kindle Book:

Juicing Recipes For Vitality And Health at Trainyourtaste.com/get-the-book

BONUS MEAL PLANS

I originally launched the first edition of this book on Amazon Kindle ebook format to get feedback from readers before publishing this physical edition. One thing that readers wanted more of were meal plans. So this next bonus section contains "FitLife approved" meals.

First, it's important to increase your fluid intake. Fluids help your body absorb vital nutrients and also help your body eliminate toxins and waste.

It is a good practice to consume 16-32 ounces of fresh juice per day in addition to eating solid foods such as vegetables and fruits. You should also be consuming 32-40 ounces of water in addition to the fresh juice.

Stay away from caffeine and alcohol since these both can dehydrate you. However, you can drink herbal teas, ginger and lemon tea, filtered water, and coconut water/almond milk.

Another tip is exercise. Make sure you at LEAST have 30 minutes of exercise per day. Remember walking is exercise.

Also if you are a vegan, you can use quinoa, brown rice and meat substitutes instead of red meat and fish.

Here is a sample weekly schedule that you can follow or modify to your tastes. More than anything, pay attention to the structure of the meals and patterns and you'll do great.

Everyday: Start out your day with drinking herbal tea or hot water with lemon and ginger. You can boil thin slices of ginger with water and then add lemon juice. It's amazing and good for you.

Day 1

Breakfast:

1 cup of steel cut oats (Choose coarse or steel cut oatmeal, since it contains more fiber. Avoid instant oatmeal, it's packed with sugar and has minimal fiber.)

- 3 cups of water

- 1/2 cup of almond milk

- cinnamon (optional)

- blueberries, strawberries (optional)

Boil 3 cups of water. Add steel cut oats to boiling water. It will take approximately 25-30 minutes to cook the steel cut oats or until the water is gone.

Once done transfer to a bowl add 1/2 cup of almond milk, cinnamon, blueberries and strawberries for taste.

Mid-morning Juice: (Remember to wait at least an hour between meals to drink fresh juice).

Green Drink

- 3 kale leaves,

- 2 collard leaves, handful of cilantro,

- 2 celery ribs,

- 1 apple,

- 2 carrots

Lunch:

- Arugula Spinach Salad with Lemon/Olive Oil Dressing

- 2 cups of arugula

- 1 cup of spinach

- 1 Avocado

- 1/2 thinly sliced red onion

- Handful of cherry tomatoes or 1 tomato cut in slices

- Dressing: Add 1 lemon, sea salt and fresh ground pepper to taste

Snack:

Handful of almonds

Mid-afternoon Juice:

"Better than a Salad Juice"

- 4 parsley springs,

- 3 tomatoes,

- 1/2 green bell pepper,

- 1/2 cucumber,

- 1 scallion,

- 1 lemon wedge.

First wrap the parsley around the tomato and add it into the juicer, then the green bell pepper, cucumber, scallion, and lemon.

Dinner:

Easy Salmon Recipe:

- Salt,

- Pepper,

- 1 tablespoon of minced fresh rosemary leaves.

- 3 lemons

- Olive oil

Serves four

Season both sides of each salmon piece with salt, pepper and rosemary leaves. Place salmon onto a piece of foil large enough to fold over. Cut 2 lemons into thin slices and place slices on salmon. Juice one lemon. Drizzle juice over salmon.

Fold over the foil and place salmon into a grill pan over medium heat for 10 minutes. Serve in foil packets.

Asparagus:

Preheat oven to 400 degrees. Bend each asparagus spear until asparagus naturally breaks. Place asparagus onto baking sheet. Drizzle olive oil over asparagus and season with small amount of salt and pepper. Place into oven for 10 minutes.

Remember to drink an adequate amount of water a total of 32 - 40 ounces.

Day 2:

Again, start out your day with herbal tea or hot water with lemon and ginger.

Breakfast:

"Beeting it with Cilantro" Juice

- 1/2 beet with green root,

- 3 carrots,

- handful of cilantro

Mid-morning snack:

Slice up an apple and drizzle cinnamon over it. It's amazing and it will fill you up.

Lunch:

- Raw Carrot Ginger Soup

- Makes 2, 1 1/2 cup servings - save 1 for dinner

- 3 cups Carrot Juice

- 1 ripe Avocado

- 1 Tbsp. Agave Nectar

- 1 Tbsp. Ginger, minced

- 1/4 tsp. ground Cayenne Pepper

- 1/4 tsp. Sea Salt

- 2 Tbsp. Fresh Cilantro

Puree the first seven ingredients in a blender until completely smooth. Taste and adjust the seasonings if necessary. Garnish the soup with a drizzle of oil and the chopped cilantro.

Mid-afternoon snack:

"Almost as Good as a Waldorf Salad Juice"

- 2 celery ribs,

- 2 green apples

Dinner

"Alpha Salad"

Make a big salad and enjoy it with a cup of raw carrot ginger soup

- 1 head of romaine hearts

- handful of cherry tomatoes

- avocado

- roasted almonds

- sliced red onions

- freshly crushed pepper

6 oz. steak (season and grill each side for 8-10 minutes depending how well done you like your steak)

Lemon and olive oil dressing: tablespoon of cold-pressed olive oil with 1 lemon and crushed pepper.

Before Bed:

Herbal tea or hot water with lemon

Day 3

Start out your day with herbal tea or hot water with lemon and ginger.

Breakfast:

Berry Delight

- 8 oz. frozen mixed berries (blueberries, raspberries and blackberries)

- steel cut oats

- almond milk

- 1 tablespoon of chopped walnuts (adds a great crunch and is packed with omega-3 fatty acids).

Boil 3 cups of water. Add 1 cup of steel cut oats. Cook for 25 - 30 minutes or until steel cut oats are cooked.

Heat the frozen berries and add it into the steel cut oats, add almond milk, add walnuts and mix ingredients together. Eat warm. It tastes like pie filling but it's very healthy.

Mid-morning Juice:

Green Juice

- 6 leaves Kale

- 2 cups Spinach

- 1/2 Cucumber

- 4 stalks Celery

- 2 Apples (fiji)

- 1" Ginger root

Lunch

- 1/2 small white onion

- 2 cloves of garlic

- 2 cups of spinach

- 1 yellow squash

- 6 oz. boneless chicken breast

- 1 teaspoon of coconut oil

- 1 teaspoon of balsamic vinegar

Add 1 teaspoon of coconut oil to saucepan or use a grill, season both sides of chicken with small amount (pinch) of freshly ground pepper. It's best to avoid salt all together.

Place chicken in saucepan or grill. Cook for 5-10 minutes on each side or until chicken breast equals 170 degrees Fahrenheit.

In a skillet add 1 teaspoon of coconut. After the coconut oil has melted thinly chop 1/2 small onion. Stir around until onion becomes transparent. Then slice 1 yellow squash and add it to the onions. Wait until squash cooks through. Stir occasionally. Add in 2 cups of spinach and cook for 5 minutes. Add 1 teaspoon of balsamic vinegar and stir. Close lid and wait 3-4 minutes. Stir again and serve!

Mid-afternoon Juice:

Original V-8 Juice Recipe

- 2 sprigs of parsley,

- 2 carrots, handful of spinach,

- 3 tomatoes,

- 3 celery ribs,

- 1/2 cucumber,

- 1/2 green bell pepper

Snack:

Handful of almonds and 1 apple

Dinner:

Vegetable Soup

- 3 Tbsp. Olive Oil

- 1 large Onion, chopped

- 3 cloves Garlic, minced

- 3 medium Carrots, chopped

- 3 Celery Stalks, chopped

- 3 Tomatoes, chopped with juice reserved

- 1 medium Zucchini, cut into half moons

- 1 cup Green Beans, trimmed to 1 inch pieces

- 3-4 handfuls Kale or other leafy green such as Chard or Bok

- Choy, chopped into small pieces

- 6 cups water

- 3/4 Tbsp. fresh Thyme, chopped

- 1 Tbsp. fresh Oregano, chopped (or 1/2 Tbsp. dried)

- 1 tsp. Sea Salt

- 1/2 tsp. fresh ground Black PepperTbsp.

In a large stock pot, heat the olive oil over medium high heat. Add the onion, garlic, carrots and celery and sauté for 5 minutes. Add the tomatoes, zucchini, green beans, water, salt, pepper, thyme and oregano; stir and bring to a boil.

Reduce the heat to a simmer and cook the soup for 10 minutes. Add the chopped kale or other leafy greens and cook for an additional 5 minutes. Season to taste with the salt and pepper.

Before bed:

Hot ginger and lemon tea

Day 4:

Remember to start out your day with herbal tea or hot water with lemon and ginger.

Breakfast

- 4 egg whites

- 1/2 steel cut oats with blueberries,

- cinnamon,

- almond milk

Mid-morning Juice:

Licorice Love

- 1 Thumb size knuckle of ginger,

- handful of mint,

- 1/2 small fennel,

- 2 apples.

Lunch:

Fitlife.tv Approved Salad

- 2 cups of chopped butter leaf lettuce

- 1 handful of walnuts

- 2 hard boiled eggs, sliced

- 1/2 avocado, sliced

- lemon and olive oil dressing with freshly ground pepper

Add ingredients to bowl and mix together

Mid-afternoon Juice:

Get Low Low Low LDL

- 1 thumb size piece of ginger,

- 1 clove of garlic,

- 4 carrots,

- 1 apple,

- splash of Tabasco sauce for an extra zing

* Wrapping the garlic in parsley helps absorb some of the garlic odor

Dinner

- 1/2 cup of brown rice (size of your fist)

- 6 oz. grilled chicken

- 2 cups of any salad greens you want

Before bed:

Hot ginger and lemon tea

Day 5

Remember to start out your day with herbal tea or hot water with lemon and ginger.

Breakfast:

- Protein Smoothie

- 1 cup of frozen berries

- 1 scoop of protein powder

- 1/2 banana

- handful of almonds

Mid-morning Juice:

Spicy Drink

- 2 large Cucumbers

- 4 cups Cilantro, leaves and stems, roughly chopped

- 1 Lime

- 1 Poblano Pepper, ribs and seeds removed

- 1 Apple

Lunch:

- 3 oz. of Alaskan Wild Salmon (If wild isn't available, get something else that is wild like halibut, white fish, or tuna. Do not buy farmed fish.)

- 1 lemon juice

- freshly ground pepper

- pinch of Himalayan salt

- 2 cups of spinach

- 1 tbsp. olive oil and lemon dressing

Season both sides of the wild salmon and place on grill of sauce pan. Cook for 10 minutes on each side. After salmon has cooked pour lemon juice over the salmon. Serve with 2 cups of spinach

Mid-afternoon Juice:

Full of Life Recipe

- 1 beet with tops,

- 1/2 medium sweet potato,

- 3 carrots

Juice beet first, then yam, then carrots.

Mid-afternoon Snack:

Handful of mixed nuts (i.e. walnuts and almonds)

Dinner

- 3 Cucumbers

- 1 tsp. Himalayan salt

- 1/2 a medium Red Onion

- 1/2 Tbsp. Ginger, finely minced

- 2 Tbsp. fresh Lime juice

- 2 Tbsp. fresh Dill, chopped

- Dash of Cayenne Pepper, optional

Peel the cucumbers and slice in half lengthwise. Place the cucumber halves cut side down on a cutting board and slice into thin half moons, about 1/4 " thick. Place in a medium sized bowl and toss with the salt. Allow the cucumbers to sit for 1 hour so that the cucumbers release some of their water. Strain the cucumbers and toss

After-Dinner Snack

Ditch the popcorn and say hello to cauliflower popcorn.

- 1 head cauliflower, cut into small florets

- 3 tablespoons olive oil

- kosher salt

- fresh crushed pepper

- 2 cloves of minced garlic

Heat oven to 400° F.

In a large bowl, combine the cauliflower, oil, and 1/2 teaspoon salt. Transfer to a baking sheet and spread in a single layer. Roast, stirring once, until golden brown and tender, about 30 minutes.

Serves 4| Hands-On Time: 10m | Total Time: 40m

Before Bed:

Hot water ginger tea with lemon.

Day 6

Start out your day with herbal tea or hot water with lemon and ginger.

Breakfast:

Scrambled Colorful Eggs

- 2 cups of spinach

- 1 cup of broccoli

- 1/2 cup of sliced read and yellow peppers

- 2 sliced cloves of garlic

- 2 eggs, 2 egg whites

- 1 small avocado

- coconut oil

- cook 2 turkey sausages (make sure they are organic)

Melt coconut oil in saucepan. Add vegetables and garlic. Then add eggs and spinach and mix together. Top off with avocado.

Morning snack:

1 apple and handful of almonds

Mid-morning Juice:

Full Immunity

- thumb size slice of ginger,

- handful parsley,

- 3 carrots,

- 1 apple

Lunch:

Original Chicken Salad

- 3 oz. chicken breast (season and grill each side for 5-10 minutes)

- 2 cups of mixed greens

- handful of cherry tomatoes

- 1/2 red bell pepper

- pinch of fresh garlic

- lemon juice, olive oil, freshly ground pepper

Mid-afternoon Juice:

Ginger Paradise Juice Recipe

- 1 thumb size slice of ginger,

- 1 apple,

- 4 carrots

Dinner:

- 6 oz. steak

- Any salad that you want

Before bed

Hot water ginger tea with lemon.

Day 7

Start out your day with herbal tea or hot water with lemon and ginger.

Breakfast:

- 4 egg whites

- 1/2 cup of steel cut oats and almond milk. Top off with cinnamon.

- 1/2 grapefruit

Mid-morning Juice

Original V-8 Juice Recipe

- 2 sprigs of parsley,

- 2 carrots, handful of spinach,

- 3 tomatoes,

- 3 celery ribs,

- 1/2 cucumber,

- 1/2 green bell pepper

Mid-afternoon snack

Handful of walnuts and 1 apple

Lunch:

- Avocado, fennel salad with grilled shrimp

- 2 tbs. of cold-pressed extra virgin olive oil

- 1 large shallot, finely diced

- 1 tsp. fennel seeds

- Himalayan salt and fresh ground pepper

- 3/4 Ib. of jumbo shrimp peeled and deveined

- 1 large head of Boston lettuce, washed and sliced into bite size pieces

- 1/2 small bulb of fennel, thinly sliced

- 1/2 cup of chopped cilantro

- 1/2 avocado

Season shrimp with olive oil, pepper and salt and grill or place in saucepan. Mix Boston lettuce with shallot, fennel, cilantro and avocado. Add shrimp and lemon and olive oil dressing and mix together.

Mid-afternoon Juice:

Detoxifying Celery Juice Recipe

- 1 cup of parsley,

- 3 carrots,

- 1 apple,

- 2 celery ribs,

- 1/2 beet with green roots.

Mid-afternoon snack

Crunch & Munch

- 2 large Carrots

- 4 stalks Celery

- 1/4 large Cucumber

- 1/2 cup Broccoli florets

- 1/2 cup Cauliflower florets

Cut carrots, celery, cucumber up into stalks. Buy a healthy, low-fat, low-sodium, dip :)

Dinner

- 2 big handfuls fresh cilantro leaves, finely chopped

- 1/2 jalapeno, sliced

- 1 teaspoon grated fresh ginger

- 1 garlic clove, grated

- 2 limes, juiced

- 2 tablespoons soy sauce

- Sea salt and freshly ground black pepper

- 1/4 cup extra-virgin olive oil

- 1 (6-ounce) block sushi-quality tuna

- 1 ripe avocado, halved, peeled, pitted, and sliced

In a mixing bowl, combine the cilantro, jalapeno, ginger, garlic, lime juice, soy sauce, salt, pepper, and 2 tablespoons of olive oil. Stir the ingredients together until well incorporated.

Place a skillet over medium-high heat and coat with the remaining 2 tablespoons of olive oil. Season the tuna generously with salt and pepper. Lay the tuna in the hot oil and sear for 1 minute on each side to form a slight crust. Pour 1/2 of the cilantro mixture into the pan to coat the fish. Serve the seared tuna with the sliced avocado and the remaining cilantro sauce drizzled over the whole plate.

Before bed

Hot water ginger tea with lemon.

Paleo Diet Resources

In this book I referred to the "Paleo" diet/lifestyle trend. I did not pioneer this diet or invent the term, but I support it as a healthy nutritional lifestyle. I also support veganism and vegetarianism as a healthy nutritional lifestyle as well... it all depends on what you want and what your body tells you it needs.

Since I barely touched on the main tenets of "Paleo" and I know some of you will wish to find more information about it, I've provided links to the following resources that you may find helpful and some of the authors that I recommend.

Listed Alphabetically By Author:

"The Paleo Diet" by Loren Cordain
http://www.amazon.com/gp/product/0470913029

"The Primal Blueprint" by Mark Sisson
http://www.amazon.com/gp/product/0982207786

"The Paleo Solution" by Robb Wolf
http://www.amazon.com/gp/product/0982565844

Claim your Free Bonus a Thank You for Reading

"Train Your Taste To Trim Your Waist."

http://www.trainyourtaste.com/reader-bonus

Made in the USA
Middletown, DE
27 March 2017